5-Minute Chi Boost

Five Pressure Points for Reviving Life Energy, Destroying Pain and Healing Fast

By

Sifu William Lee

Author of Amazon Bestsellers

Healing Chi Meditation

Total Chi Fitness

T.A.E. Total Attack Elimination

5-Minute Stress Management

Chi Healing Powers Book Set

Total Self Defense Book Set

ACKNOWLEDGMENTS

To my students and friends. You are all selflessly helping me.

Special thanks to those who asked, insisted and assisted me in turning the seminars in to this practical form.

CONTENTS

CUSTOMER REVIEWS

By John Parson

The book is not that long, but there is some really great information in it. I have been dong the qigong exrcises in it for about 2 weeks now and have had great results. Yesterday at work I was just about to fall asleep and decided to do the exercise, what an energy boost that was! Anyone wanting to have a simple way to get a lot of energy real fast and a lot of other health benefits should buy this book.

By Michael D. Lawrience

If we choose we all can take 5 minutes a day to improve our health. Opening up our meridians and acupressure points provides an effective way.

The author gives the specifics with diagrams for boosting your liver, kidney, and other meridians. I like that he gives a system so you can see how many times a day you need to do the 5 exercises.
I have over 35 years experience as an energy healer. I have used most of these methods 1, 2, 4, and 5. They work.

Buy this book now and use these simple and effective methods. Develop the discipline. Take the time to improve your health and well-being.

By Dr.Johns

I am myself an experienced MD and have published a guide about acupressure. And, from an expert point of view, I can honestly say this is an awesome book and very much recommended. It is very easy to follow even for the newbie, and it make this science easily reachable for everybody. The only negative thing I found is that it's kind of short, too much straight to the point. But if you are really short of time, and you are concerned about improving your health, then this book is just what you need.

INTRODUCTION:

Do You Need This Program?

Honestly, I can't tell you whether or not you need this program – but I can help answer this question quickly. The first thing you should know is that this isn't a theoretical work with piles of data and information. It is entirely focused on practical methods that can easily revive your energy levels, help you heal and stay healthy. This program is the fruit of my lifelong dedication to studying traditional Chinese forms of healing. Among the healing methods and practices (I refer only to genuine and effective ones), this is probably one of the easiest ones for learning, and probably the quickest to apply. Besides that:

-Its potency is not watered down in any way.
-You do not need anything else in order to receive the full benefit from this simple yet powerful program.
-You can easily show these methods to your children, friends or anyone in need.

If you are experiencing any of the below-listed symptoms and needs, the 5-Minute Chi Boost with simple pressure point stimulation methods will definitely help you, and probably answer the "do you need this book" question!

- Lack of energy

- Suffering from headaches
- Difficulties in maintaining focus
- Feelings of physical or mental weakness
- Desire to increase weight loss results
- Desire to improve detoxing results
- Suffering from any chronic pain
- Suffering from allergies
- Difficulty enjoying life without painkillers and/or medication
- High or low blood pressure issues
- Suffering from a digestion disorder
- Want to speed up healing time from illness or after surgery
- Desire to prevent chronic "sick and tired" feelings
- Need to boost your libido and sex drive or
- you simply want a boost for your energy levels and performance

I am not saying these simple practices are the 'ultimate solution for all problems of this world'. This is not a 'magic pill', and sometimes it's necessary to look at complex programs that are aimed at particular health disorders.

My next book will give an in-depth explanation of all aspects of the Chi Kung art (you can visit my chi power blog (www.chi-powers.blogspot.com) for news about the release date and other useful information). In fact, you will simply be blown away once you start applying this 5-Minute Chi Boost program.

CHAPTER ONE: WHY THIS BOOK?

We Are All Longing for …

People differ from each other in many ways. However, every individual is the same color on the inside. Whatever lifestyle we choose, regardless of how that is perceived by those around us (attractive, beneficial, stupid or even repulsive) - any combination of actions that form something we call "lifestyle" is essentially aimed at achieving the same goal.

Without attaining "it", life doesn't make much sense. If we don't experience "it" for longer periods of time, we lose a desire to even get up in the morning. We all are striving for happiness! You can label it differently, you can hunt for it by involving yourself in various (material or spiritual) activities but at the end of the day, the fact remains: human beings are in constant search for happiness and bliss. We all are trying hard to "earn happiness" or just feel happy! If we didn't have that "pleasure-hunting" instinct deeply rooted in our programing, then why would people go through trials and tribulations just to raise their quality of life? For what other "ultimate gain" would anyone desire to have more money, to graduate from a University or (for the sake of argument) go through the pain of plastic surgery? What is the reason that we prefer to be near "it" and we strongly avoid something else? No one likes to feel sick and weak because ultimately, the feeling of happiness and bliss is what we all are "dying for". Now, this book is not about life philosophy. It is not about meditation, religion or anything like that. I promise, this book will offer you very simple and practical methods that will assist you to faster in attaining….

- Happiness in life

No one wants …

We all know that a person can't enjoy almost any aspect of life when exposed to disease or pain. Going through any sort of pain quickly destroys our natural ability to enjoy what life offers. Did you know that there is a condition that appears before any sort of pain, diseases and disorder? It is simpler than you can imagine right now. My dear friend, that condition very much exists, it is very real. In simple words we can call it the 'weak flow of Chi' (life energy). Regardless of the name we decide to use (Prana, Chi, aura, electromagnetic bio field, Ki or some other name), we do speak about the same energy – energy of life. It is the energy that pervades all that exists and everything around us.

It is very important for you to understand this fact: reviving a naturally strong, healthy flow of Chi is a way to avoid pain and disease simply because weak Chi flow develops before any type of disorder manifests. (Please note: The methods that I explain in this 5-Minute Chi Boost book are not meant only for those already suffering from poor health.)

"Noah's Ark was build before the heavy rain started"!

Without a tinge of pessimism (only keeping in mind the way most people live today), I am pretty sure life will "start raining" even if you feel full of energy and you enjoy perfect health. The aim of this publication is the demystifying and teaching about powerful yet simple methods to strengthen the flow of Chi (life energy) of a body. In the ancient Chinese art of Chi Kung, as well as traditional Chinese martial arts, Chi has been nourished in a natural way for centuries. Here, I explain some of the most effective methods that you can start benefiting from very quickly. Once you revive your healthy and strong flow of energy, you not only regain your natural healthy state, but also you make sure that no physical (or mental) disorder will become part of your life experience, ever again. (Some of the best things in life seem to be "too simple", right?) It all depends on individual decisions - if you take a bit of your time to learn these powerful "5-Minute Chi Booster" methods you will eventually reap the benefits of living without …

- **Disease and Pain**

You Don't Need Much of …

Over the years, I noticed that only a few individuals dedicate much time for seriously exploring subjects that I lecture about. Most people do not have much time. Many people have attended my seminars and courses on Acupressure, Meridian Therapy, Self

Defense and Chi Kung over the years. Even in the early 1980's, I clearly remember that time pressure was a problem, it's what most of us experience, and it's one of the crucial reasons I actually started changing the way I teach. I am blessed to have wonderful people willing to assist me in molding the style of my teaching. It works well for my seminars and courses and I believe it will show the same effect in this book.

This 5-Minute Chi Booster program is simple and powerful, yet (as the name suggests) it is not a demanding, time-intensive subject to learn and apply. In order to master the techniques in this book you don't need a lot of ….

- **Time**

CHAPTER 2: CHI – IMPORTANT FACTS

As I have promised, this book is not a theoretical pile of information, but let's review the most important characteristic related to 'life force'.

As you probably know, ancient manuscripts originating in different cultures offer explanations on various subject matters related to manipulating life force. Despite my dedication to 'energy work', naturally I couldn't find time to study all of the traditions. However, from what I have read I do understand the following: all traditions understand the subject of 'energy that powers all that leaves' in a fairly similar way, though some are focused on certain aspects that I do not see as very useful and practical for today.

Let's have a quick look at those facts that are important to know for success with the 5-Minute Chi Boost Program. If you are already a student of any related practice, and you don't consider yourself a newbie due to the knowledge that you have already acquired, feel free to skip over these first few lines. I'm well aware that these may sound simple to some of you. On the other hand, I've experienced that it's never wrong to go over the basics. Many readers will find some of these facts very helpful, even if they have knowledge in this area. Here is short summary of most important fact about Chi:

- Chi (also written as 'Qi') is a vital force of energy and life present throughout the material creation, and without its presence, no symptom of life can be seen.

- Chi, or ‘energy of life’ or ‘life force’, is named differently in various philosophies and cultures (Ki in Japan, Prana in Indian Vedas, Mana in Hawaiian culture, Lüng in Tibetan Buddhism etc.) yet all those sources of knowledge speak about the same vital energy.

- As in nature, Chi is constantly circling and flowing in our bodies, supplying life force to each and every limb, muscle and organ.

- Chi travels through the body using subtle energy channels known as 'meridians'. There are many main energy centers and pressure points situated along these energy paths.

- Whenever a healthy flow of Chi is disturbed or it weakens, the body develops a certain pain or disease in order to bring our attention to the source of a problem.

- By proper treatment using various pressure points, breathing and posture, one can efficiently revive the healthy and strong flow of a ‘life force’ in our bodies. That is the essence of health.

- This knowledge is not difficult to master nor it is reserved for some special group of people. Everyone who decides can successfully learn the 5-Minute Chi Boost techniques regardless of beliefs, age, education, sex or any other material condition.

These are, in my experience, basic and most important facts we have to know about. As with other areas of study, it's only a question if the individual really decides to do something about that knowledge or not. When we really decide to do/have/experience 'something', sooner or later we will end up doing/having/experiencing exactly that. Therefore, my only question to you is:

'Are you serious about improving your health and well-being?'

Now, allow me to request you to stop reading further. Before continuing just answer this question, please. If you are alone in the room, you can even say it. If you have a mirror nearby (a mobile camera option could work just fine), even better - just look deep into your own eyes and simply answer on this question. No one else needs to hear your answer but you! This is very important. Want to know why? Well, I have to be honest with you. You really need to be clear about the answer on that question above because these techniques, which I'm going to teach here, generate one problem. If your answer is "Yes" and you are fully clear about that, you will be able to overcome that problem. Otherwise, I am not sure that you can …

CHAPTER 3: PROBLEM SOLVED

Though I cannot be sure you will experience this problem, in my experience, most people who decide to try out this 5-Minute Chi Boost program are faced with it - though the majority of students go through it and experience the best effects later. We do not want any blockages, especially when you learn how effective this program really is. So, what is the problem with the 5-Minute Chi Boost?

In short, the 'problem' is that the techniques of this program are just too effective for our Western mindsets! Results do appear fast in various forms such as relief from pain, a feeling of freshness, better ability to concentrate, etc. All of that is very appealing – which is why it can be a 'problem' and a reason to be a bit more prepared. Life becomes enjoyable again, and as a result, some people just stop the program entirely too soon!

One has to know a bit more about 5-Minute Chi Boost potency in order derive the maximum benefit from it. If you stop this program too soon, the Chi flow revival circle will not be completed fully. In case of light and easy health disorders, that is NOT a big problem because those are normally solved fast or, if the symptoms come back, one can just start with the program again.

However, in case of deep-rooted health problems,

closing the full Chi flow revival circle is needed. I will give you the recommended formula right now - it is actually very simple. Just follow it and you will find yourself on the safe side. Here is the *'full problem solved'* 5-Minute Chi Boost formula.

1. Read this book and start the program.

2. Note the start date in your calendar, scheduler or mobile phone.

3. When you notice that your main pain / negative symptom is completely gone, note how many days have passed.

4. Continue doing the 5-Minute Chi Boost program for **at least** the same time period. Just do it every day, you won't be sorry.

<u>Let me give you few real life examples:</u>

- Jessica R. (age 41, working as Post Office clerk, divorced four years, 2 kids) started with the 5-Minute Chi Boost program due to chronic tiredness and migraines. After 3 weeks of "not religiously doing 5-Minute Chi", she characterized her problems as 80-90% gone. After 5 weeks she emailed me with "the last time I felt so good was a long time ago. Headache is completely gone and I can normally function without prescription meds and energy drinks again…" I recommended her to go on with 5-Minute

Chi Boost for the next 5 weeks.

- Tiffany M. (age 56, housewife, living an active lifestyle, married, 4 children). She started with the 5-Minute Chi Boost program to speed up her post-surgery recovery. In her own words, "…low energy level and weakness of body and will.." were main reasons to give the 5-Minute Chi a try. In the first 10 days of "…doing 3 sets every morning and 2 sets in the evenings" she characterized her problems as 50% gone. 7 weeks after the start, she reported this: "…I honestly could not imagine something as simple as this could have such a profound effects on my condition. In answer to your questionnaire I can say that I am now 99% better – 1% is still hanging around like a bad smell in a room…." I recommended her to go on with the 5-Minute Chi Boost for the next 7 – 8 weeks after that.

- Adrian W. (age 37, manager in real estate agency, married, 2nd marriage, 2 kids from 1st marriage, 1 kid in 2nd marriage, history of drug / alcohol abuse, 4 years clean). Adrian took my Complete Chi Kung Revival seminar (the topic of my next book) but decided to go with the 5-Minute Chi Boost program due to a 'very busy schedule'. The main problems he pointed out were: "…lack of energy to keep up with all I have to do….I do suffer from weak libido….I really am annoyed due to my difficulties in concentration (especially after lunch)…" Two weeks after switching to "…. doing 2 cycles of your Chi Boosting in the morning and almost every evening one cycle…." Adrian emailed me with a 95% 'problems gone' message. Despite my knowledge about inner potency that methods in this program hold, I had to make sure that he is realistic about this.

Long story short, 4 weeks after the start with the program he reported "I would never waste my and your time. After all the c*****p I have done to my self in my life, I am now more than careful with what I do or not do. Respected Sifu Lee, be sure I am a new man, I am cured...." I recommended him a minimum of 21 days with the same pace of the 5-Minute Chi Boost routine.

You should now have a clear understanding about how things work and how to use the *'full problem solved'* 5-Minute Chi Boost formula. It's really as simple as that. Naturally, you have to be realistic and honest when assessing your success.

<u>Word of caution:</u> there is no need to e-mail me with the results or to 'depend' on me for any further guidance. Students that I personally trained give the above examples, and the reports were a planned element of that step-by-step personal training.

Also, I think you would be happy to hear the following. Those students were not equipped with all of the detailed explanations, guidelines and photographs in concise written material, like you have in your hands right now! This book had not yet been written and I did not use any written materials before. I have started writing this book in order to achieve a better quality of teaching. Naturally there are positive aspects of personal teaching, but the beauty of a book is that you can always re-read if you are not sure about something. In that way, you will definitely get the most out of this program.

CHAPTER 4: FIVE PRESSURE POINT METHODS

This practical part is the main and most critical part of this book. If you get to understand the methods described here in this chapter only (and you put them in to practice), you will definitely get the same benefits as a person who reads this book from beginning to end. The reason for that is very simple. The techniques from the 5-Minute Chi Boost formula are mainly the pressure point treatments. The same as all other unchanged approaches I teach about, if explained properly and correctly, they are not subjective or questionable - they simply work regardless of the outside world and its influences.

On top of that, you can have faith in Chi 'power' or you can be a total Chi agnostic, but if you apply everything properly you will get the results. Now, another problem that I see sometimes is that people expect to get the best results without doing things properly. That will not work. The same as with anything else in this world, you won't get the full results if you make a partial effort or if you do things the wrong way. These five pressure point stimulation methods are simple to learn and apply. You only have to learn them and apply them as recommended every day, or simply any time you feel weak, tired and in need of a powerful Chi Boost. Because there are just too many effects and indications of every method this program contains, I won't list every benefit you get below each method - it would take up too much space.

(For an overview, you can always read the list at the beginning of the book. This program has the power to help you fight and defeat each of those.)

Before we start, here is short disclaimer. You have to consult your physician before starting this program. Do not start doing these exercises if you have any of the following conditions:

- Pregnant (11 weeks or more) or lactating.
- Open wounds or new injuries (just after an accident and still swelling, inflammation and fractures, or right after any sort of surgery).
- Cardiac Pacemaker.

PREPARATION

Before you start with the 5-Minute Chi Boost, it is good to know about things that will accelerate your results.

Breathing:

Before you start, it's good to calm down and bring fresh oxygen in to system. This is easily done when you breathe deeply for a few minutes. You can do simple pranayama or abdominal breathing exercises. If you have not been introduced to those, here is the quickest course on therapeutic breathing you will ever see:

- If you are not outside, arrange to have fresh air in a room.
- Sit or stand up comfortably with your spine straight.
- Touch your upper palate with your tongue.
- Breathe in through your nose, and breathe out through your mouth.
- While you breathe in, start pushing your abdomen out (so that the down part of your lungs become active and involved).
- Continue filling your lungs with air (middle part to the upper lungs).
- Exhale in opposite order: start emptying your upper lungs first, then the middle, all the way to your abdomen.

For those who want to learn more, my next book will teach you a lot more about Chi breathing, but this are the basics and it all starts from right here. I advise breathing deeply, not only as preparation, but also the entire time while doing the 5-Minute Chi Boost exercises.

Time:

Best times for doing them are in the morning (immediately after you wake up) and around 3 p.m. due to the phases and positions of (Yin and Yang) energies in a body. Alternatively, you can do them in the evening (2 hours or more before going to sleep), or whenever you feel you need a fresh boost of energy.

Cycles:

5-Minute Chi Boost exercises are done in cycles. You start with the 1st exercise, then 2nd, 3rd, 4th and when you are over with the 5th, there is your first cycle - done. In beginning, (maybe the first few times) it may take a bit longer, but as soon as you learn these simple methods, it shouldn't take you longer than 5 minutes to perform one full Chi Boost cycle.

'Dosage':

How many cycles you should do is very individual, depending on your health issues and how 'bad' you desire to feel better. Don’t worry - I won't leave you hanging with only that . Here is how to decide on a perfect 'dosage' that will best suit your situation. Answer this question to yourself right now.

The _________ (condition / health problem) that I am suffering from, disturbs my natural ability to enjoy in life by ______%

Grade it on a scale of 1 to 100 % (1 = hard to even feel and 100 = impossible to tolerate). Below are recommended cycles according to how disturbed you feel:

- 1-25% - minimum 1-3 cycles of 5-Minute Chi Boost exercises a day
- 25-50% - minimum 3-9 cycles of 5-Minute Chi Boost exercises a day*
- 50+% - 3 times a day (morning, 3pm, evening), 5 cycles*

One cycle is obviously a minimum. Please note that I do not recommend **anyone** doing more than 5 cycles (~25 minutes) of 5-Minute Chi Boost exercises at one time.

*If your answer is 50% or more, please note this: 5-Minute Chi Boost program is very powerful but you need to do more for your health! Get a complete holistic healing program that you prefer. Also, you must see your physician and consult with him.

Use this 5-Minute Chi Boost program to accelerate

your healing speed and potency. It will help you more than you think.

I: Energy Slapping

This is a method (as the name suggests) that is applied by slapping. It is aimed on the main meridians on the body and pressure points situated all over them. You have to use your palms to apply stimulation to areas of your body as shown below. Use your palms fully, not just your fingers.

The Key Element of Energy Slaps (most people do not get these right) is appropriate strength. Slapping has to be strong and firm, not too soft or weak. The photograph can show you the position, but you have to understand this. Just use your common sense here.

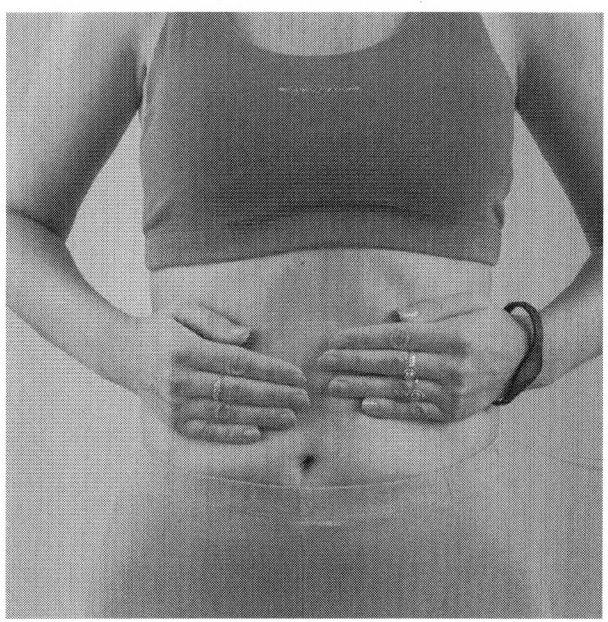

It's all about having a healthy balance, same as in most (or all) things in life, right? Enough power to feel it, not too much power so that you are in pain. You do not need a masochistic approach here □ because anytime you go over the edge of pain, the body puts up a defense reaction that "closes up" the meridians even more … and you don't want that to happen.

i. Points we start with are on each side of the central line of the abdomen and stomach. Start on a level of the pubic bone and slowly move up. There are 4 'levels' you want to work on, 2 times on each point – the last one you should treat 3 times. That is nine times (slapping's) in total; remember that number and you will do yourself a favor.

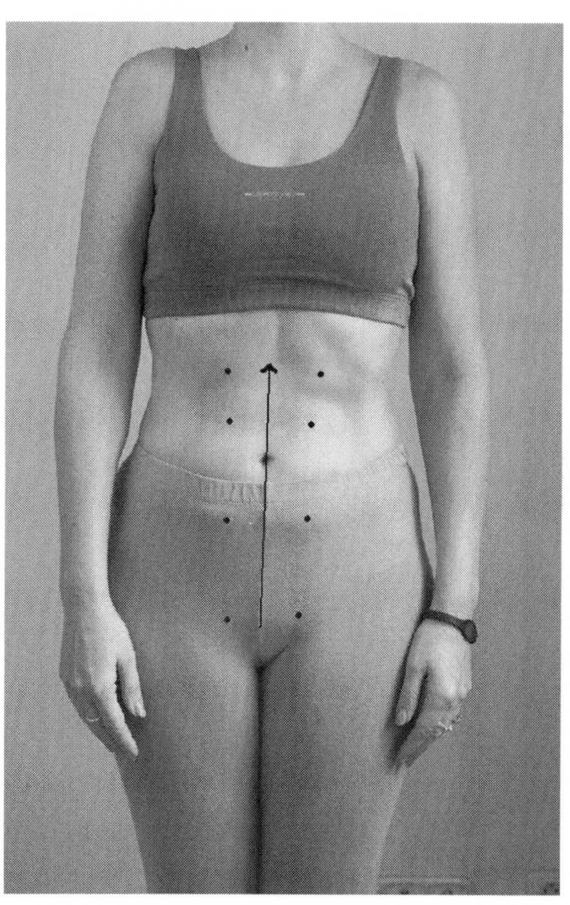

ii. Starting with your left hand, (women should start from just above the breast on a left) slap over the right side of the chest area, diagonally up to the middle of the trapezius muscle - 9 times.

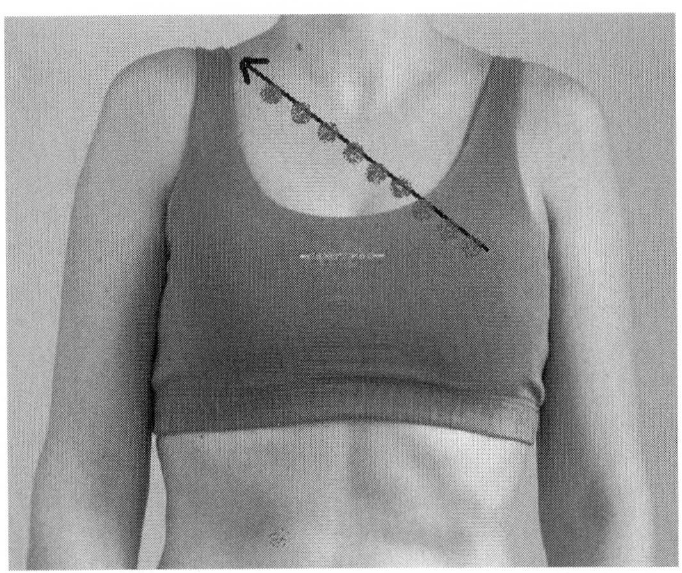

iii. Keep slapping on top of the trapezius muscle, exactly in the middle - 9 times - you should feel the striking up all the way down in your legs, just don't overdo it (normally it is pleasant to slap bit harder on this point).

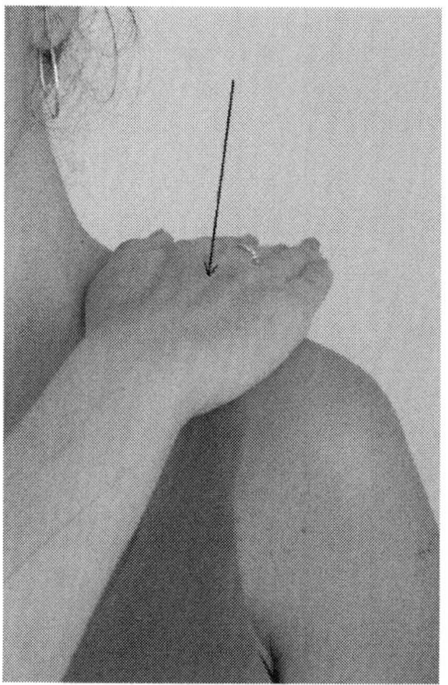

iv. Move across your right shoulder, upper arm, forearm and wrist, all the way to the upper (back) side of your palm. (Just to make sure we are on the same page, we treat the left side of the body first, **then** the right side). So, moving slowly across the arm, double the amount - this area needs ~18 slaps.

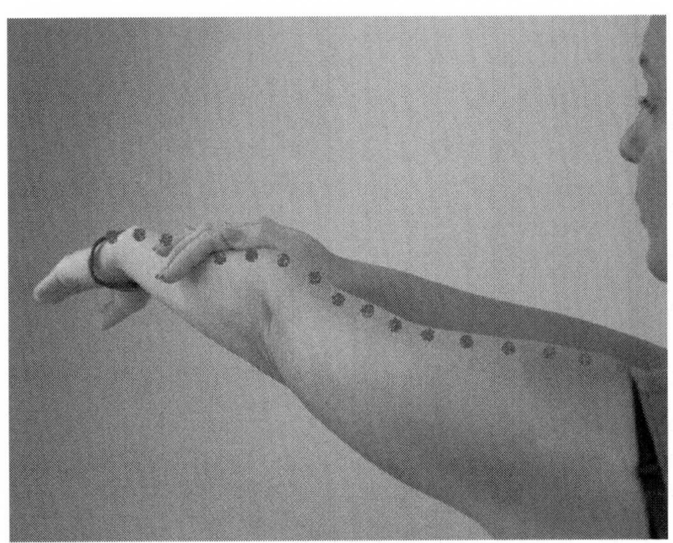

v. Turn your palm upwards and apply the same 18 slaps now on the inner side of the arm, moving in the opposite direction. Same as on the upper side, the inner side of the arm holds many important pressure points, because there are 3 meridians positioned on each side of the arm. However, for most people the inner side of the arm is a bit more sensitive to pain, so keep that in mind.

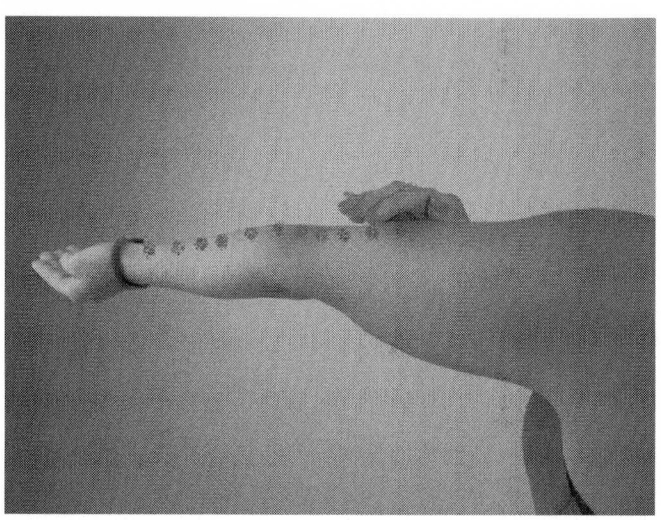

On the photograph, the last few points are not visible. It's important that you follow the inner side toward your armpit – as simple as that.

vi. Once you reach the armpit, work on it for duration of 9 slaps.

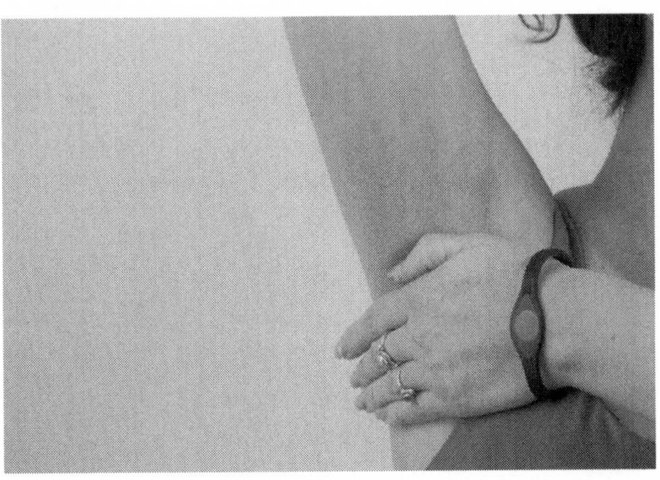

This is very beneficial to all parts, but this part has an incredibly strong influence on female bodies. It is proven to be a safe prevention from breast cancer. (I promised we'd keep it practical - let's move on.)

vii. Next is the step ii. now aimed in opposite direction: you simply slap the pressure points down, from the collarbone area, to where you have started in step ii. diagonally across the chest.

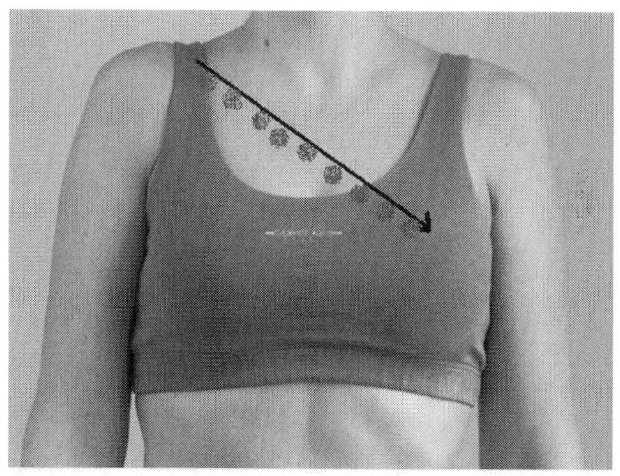

viii. NEXT, you have to switch to another side of your body. Using your right palm, simply repeat steps ii. - vii. - That's important. Never treat only one side of your body.

ix. Now you are back to using both palms. This is same as in step i. but now from up downwards, from the ribcage down to the pubic bone – apply three Chi slaps to the first level, and all others two times so it's 3 + 2 + 2 + 2 = 9 slaps in total.

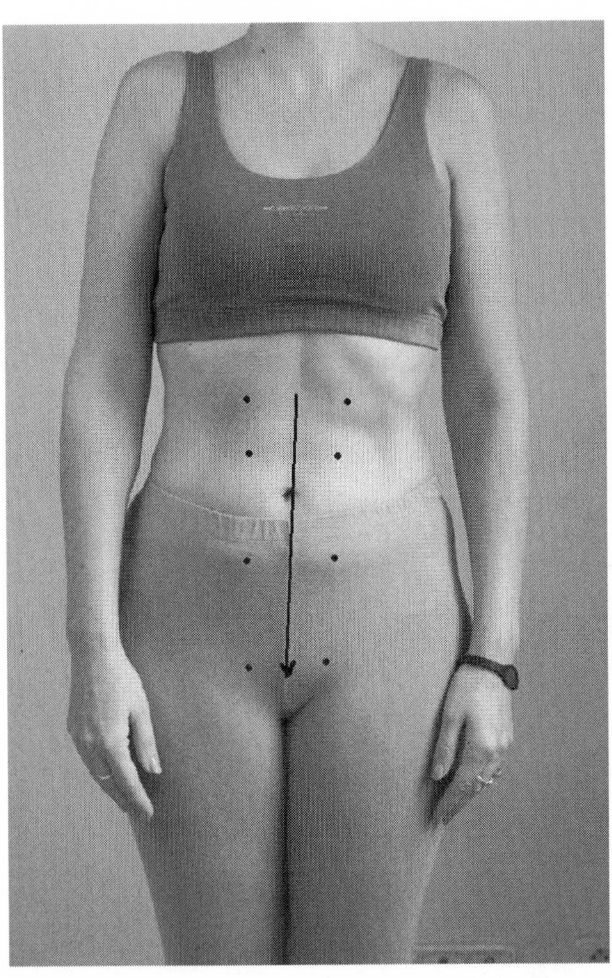

x. Move palms to your hips. Here, on the legs, some people do feel "more pain" but since bodies differ some need to use more power in order to feel anything. It really depends, have that in mind.

From the hips, you move down to your feet using the outer side of the legs. Legs are longer than arms, so you can do from 18 up to 27 slaps. Stop on your ankles and switch to the next exercise.

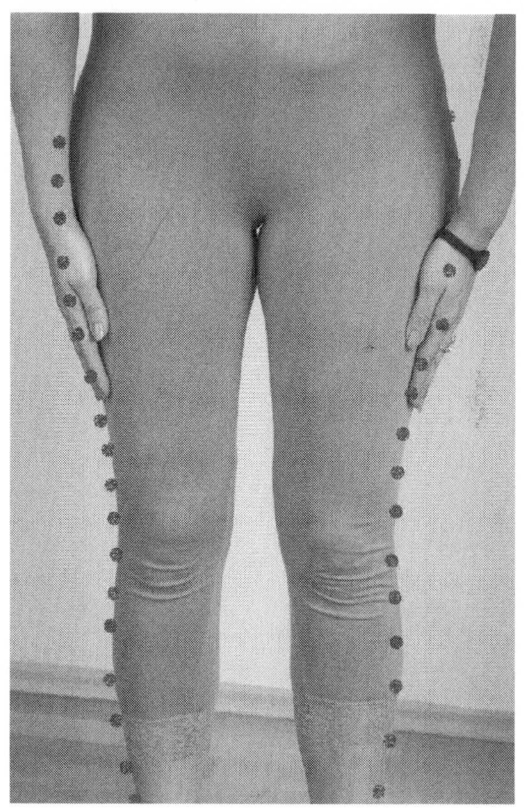

xi. Once down on the ankles, switch to the inner side of the legs and move straight upward. This area is normally sensitive yet I have seen people that do not feel much here and need to apply with power even in this area. Apply 18 to 27 slaps.

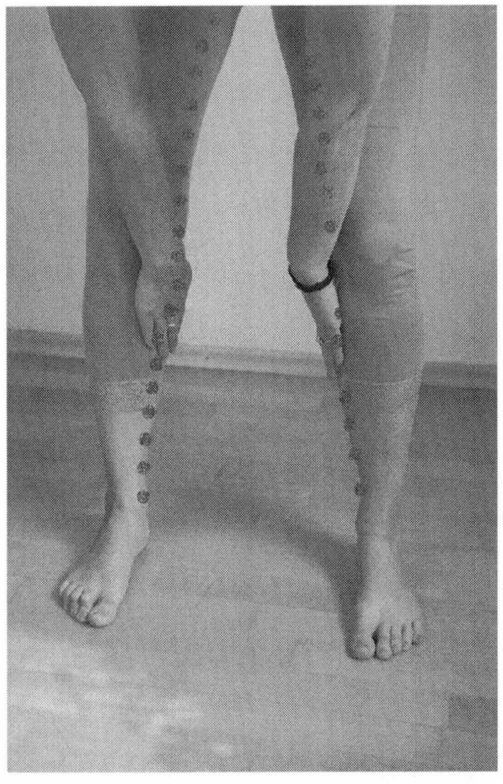

That is the end of the Energy Slapping exercise method. It covers the main meridians of the body, and will wake up 'sleepy' Chi and make it flow strongly trough your internal organs (and your energy centers as well), which will refresh your body and mind for a fast track to healing.

NOTE: Breathe deeply the entire time during all parts of the Energy Slapping cycles, and have your tongue touching the upper palate.

II: Feet 1 (Tai-Chan)

This is one of the main pressure points used for revitalizing the body, detoxification, easing pains, etc. Seriously, there are so many things to be said about Tai-Chan – a separate chapter for each of these exercises would be needed for one who wants to study them in depth. Since at this time we are all about practical and quick results...

i. Locate the Tai-Chan point on your feet. Between your big toe and middle toe, there is a soft tissue area. Tai-Chan is situated about 1.5 inches downwards. If you use your thumb, you can't miss it. It is a sensitive point. Just apply the pressure across that line and you will know exactly when you hit the right spot, no doubt (ouch!).

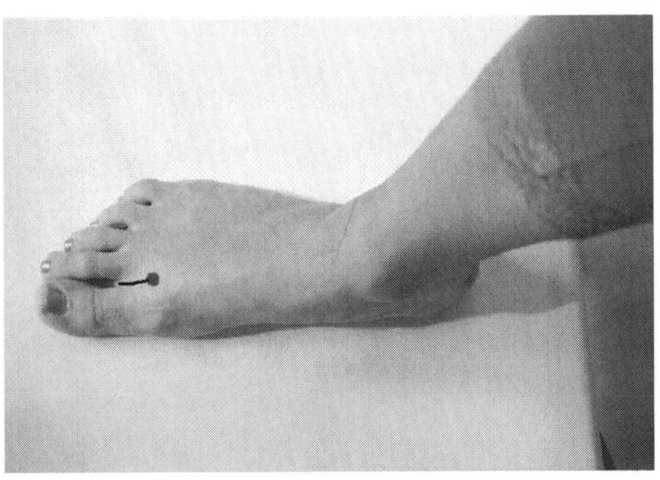

ii. Best here to use is called the 'double thumb' pressure. Put one thumb over another, and apply pressure. Again, this is a sensitive pressure point - pain here has to be of a 'pleasant nature'. Never cross over the edge of your pain tolerance.

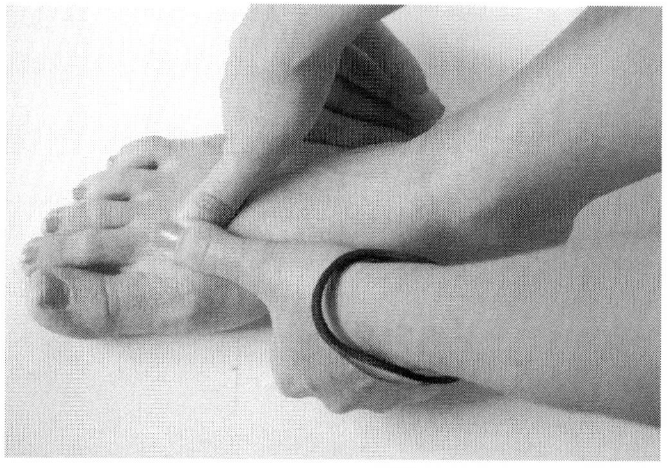

iii. Keep pressing for 9 seconds, and repeat 3 times. Take a short 2-3 second break between repetitions.
iv. Repeat the same on the right side.
v. Breathe deeply the entire time while treating the Tai-Chan pressure point and have your tongue touching the upper palate.

That's it. We move to the next powerful pressure point that will force Chi to circle even more.

III: Feet 2 (Yang-Quan)

This pressure point is located a bit deeper inside your body tissues. You will probably have to apply more pressure. Without any further explanations, this is our next pressure point:

i. Locating the Yang-Quan point: below the thumb, there is a fleshy part. When you move pressure on its inner edge, just a bit below the ending, you will feel a small depression. It's not difficult to locate Yang-Quan as it is sensitive as well.

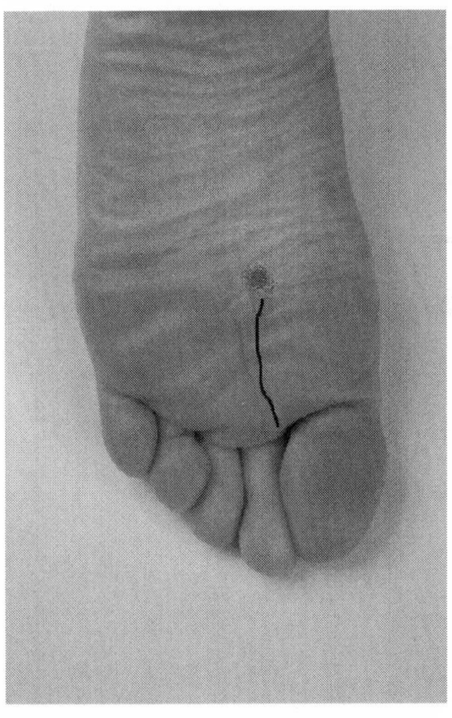

ii. Apply the pressure with thumb or with fingertips.

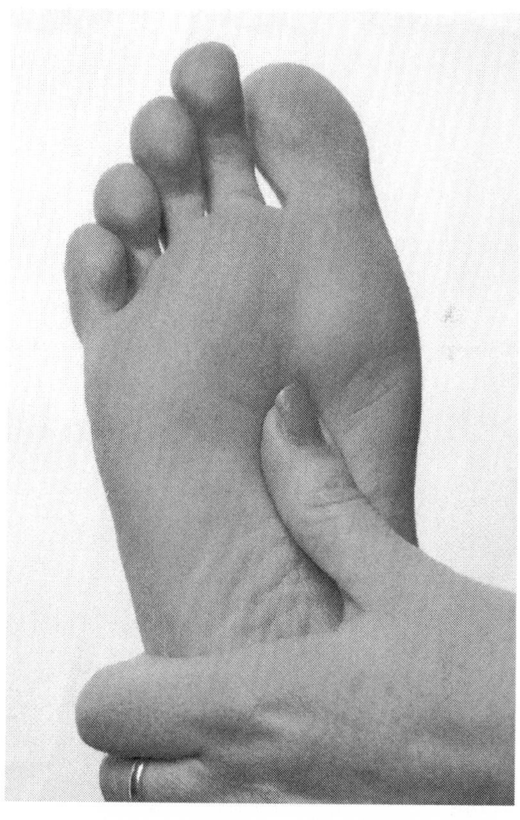

iii. Keep pressing for 9 seconds, and repeat that 3 times. Take a short 2-3 second break between repetitions.
iv. Repeat the same on the right foot.
v. You can use any sort of pressure applied by the tips of your fingers. It is not necessary to use the thumb.

vi. Breathe deeply the entire time while doing Yang-Quan, and have your tongue touching the upper palate.

IV: Kidney Boost

This kidney area has great importance for general health, the immune system and other vital functions of the body. We'd better just skip to the practical part, there is just too much to be said about the importance of these pressure points. I fully believe you know how to locate your kidney area □ but in order to be sure, this is the area I would ask you to massage / rub (in the whole area, not just the pressure point):

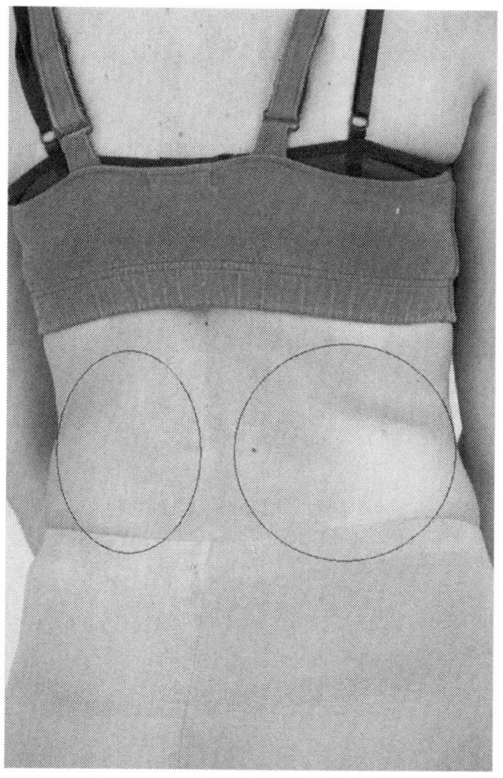

Pay attention, please: - we have a "new" element to apply BEFORE we do a Kidney Boost. Again, it is a simple thing but it has to be done properly. Here is *what* and *how* to do it:

i. Rub your palms together for at least 30 seconds and keep your focus and attention there. Pleasant heat will be generated fast, that is what we need.

ii. Keep rubbing your palms until you feel a good amount of heat there.

iii. Put your (warmed) palms on the kidney area and start rubbing both the left and right sides of the kidney area, using both hands.

iv. Do that for at least 45 seconds, gradually increasing the pressure and intensity.

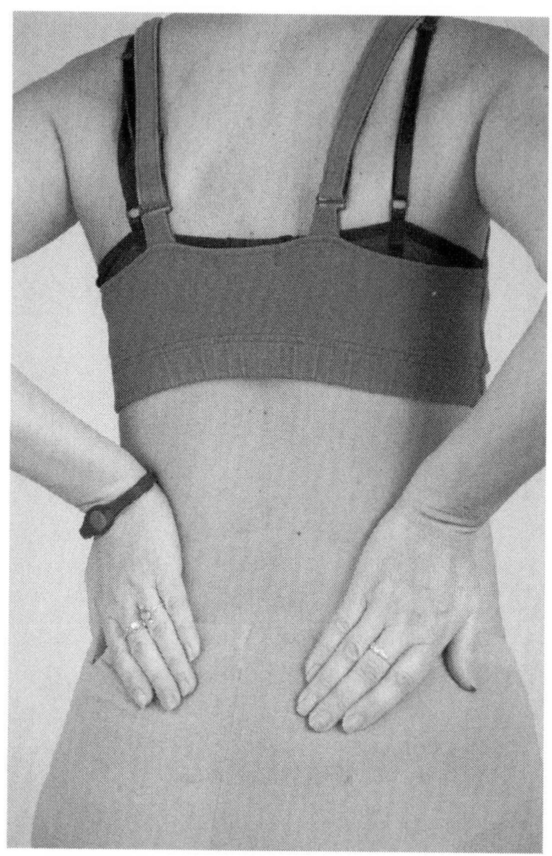

v. Breathe deeply the entire time, and have your tongue touching the upper palate.

V: Triple Power Tapping

This one is the last practical part of this program. It consists of treating three very potent pressure points. Here are few more details about Triple Power Tapping:

- You perform tapping with your fingertips, joined together
- It's not a gentle tap but quite strong "striking" on the chosen areas.
- Don't torture yourself, but you have to feel that this is really 'good'.

Thymus Boost:

i. Locate your chest bone.
ii. Start by tapping the middle part of the chest bone. Slowly move your tapping upwards to the collarbone level where the chest bones ends.
iii. Tap 18 times.
iv. Breathe deeply the entire time, and have your tongue touching the upper palate.

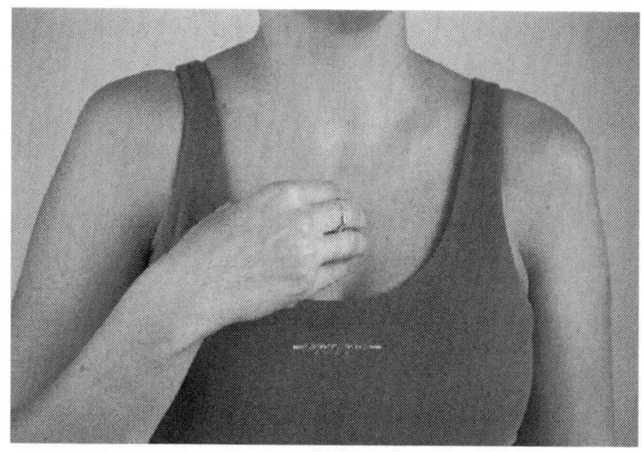

K-27:

This is pressure point number 27 on the kidney meridian, a very powerful pressure point. Many people (even those serious about Chi Kung, Acupressure etc.) cover K27 in their books and programs.

I think the main reasons are:

- It's not very easy to find K27, but it's not hard either. You can locate it quickly in the following way:

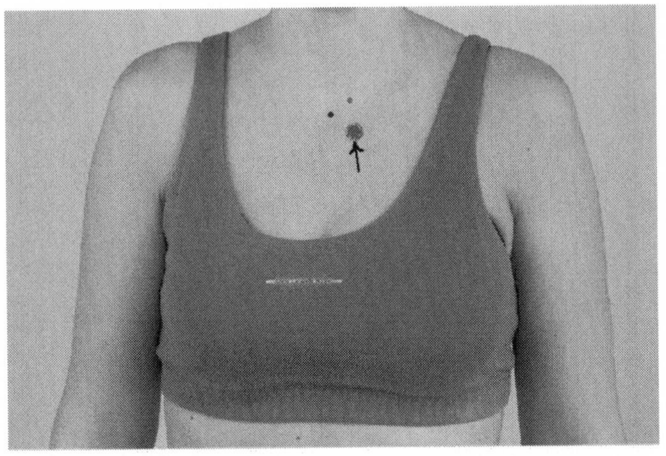

- Another reason is the upper chest muscles may 'block' access to K-27 in those (men especially) with more developed chest muscles. If you are in that group, just do one left side first, then the right. When your arm is down, the upper chest muscles will stay out of your way.

i. Put your finger in the hole between the collarbones (blue point).

ii. Find the corner / beginning of the collarbone (pink point).

iii. Move down a across your collarbone diagonally and find the 'fleshy' part just bellow the collarbone edge. If you apply enough pressure, you will feel this pressure point quickly (ouch again □).

iv. Tap it firmly 18 times left side then right OR do both sides at the same time.

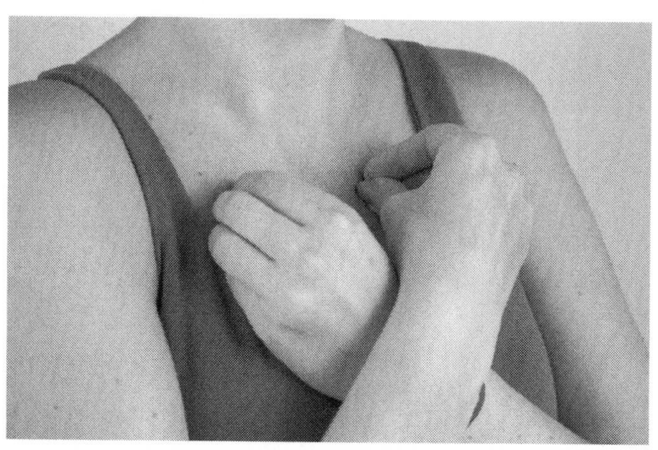

v. Breathe deeply the entire time, and have your tongue touching the upper palate.

<u>'Rib Side' Energy</u>: There are a few sensitive pressure points in this area, so it's important that you find and treat exactly this one. Another few points located in a same line (meridian) are also potent, but not as much as this one. Do not worry; you can't harm yourself even if you miss.

However, you can't miss if you follow my guideline, you will get it right.

i. This point is located in a half-moon shaped line under the line of the breast.

ii. When you put your arms into position like in the photograph, your fists will be positioned exactly under these points.

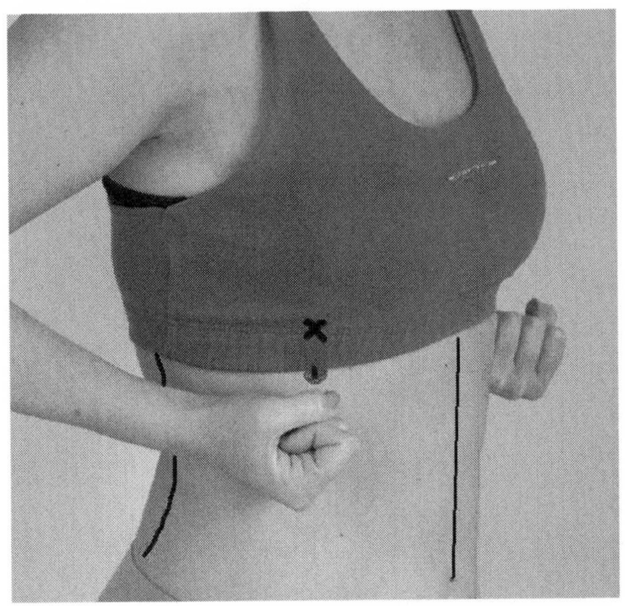

iii. To be sure you locate the correct point, apply pressure by finger across the half-moon shaped line below the breast (the lower edge of women's bras goes almost exactly over that line).

iv. Keep your pressure steady and the 'Rib Side' Energy pressure point will let you know (yes, ouch again □) as soon you get on it.

v. Tap firmly 18 times both sides at the same time.

vi. Breathe deeply the entire time, and have your tongue touching the upper palate.

Rely on your body and its reaction. Once you locate it, you have to keep your fingertips together, focused on applying strong (and balanced) tapping.

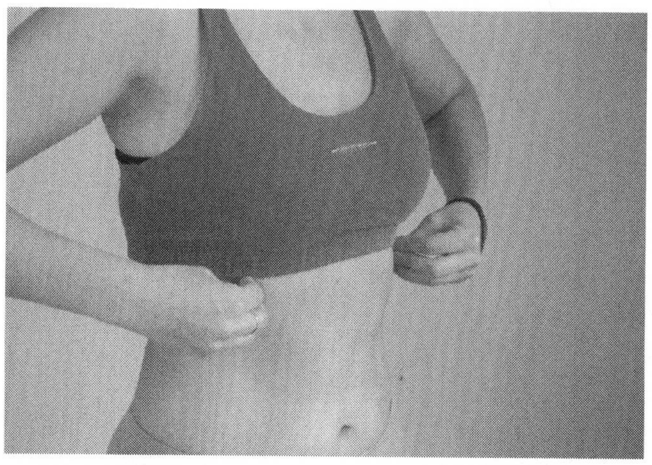

This photograph (and other photos presented here) will assist and help you to learn these methods quickly. Please keep this in mind: different human bodies have different constitutions, so the visual position of this and other pressure points won't look the same on all bodies. However that's not a problem. Body and mind will reveal the exact locations of all pressure points you need, when you start following the simple guidelines given herein.

You can get the videos of all exercises right from this link here, http://eepurl.com/OZgZj. Please subscribe to a list, confirm your email and allow up to 1hour time and you will get email with the links to videos. We will NOT spam, sell or misuse your email in any way, do not worry.

If you cant click on the link and land on subscription page, please type this URL in to your browser http://eepurl.com/OZgZj

NOTE: NEED MORE POWER?

5-Minute Chi Boost methods remained unchanged thousands of years and they will for sure help you, there is no doubt about this. However, we are all individuals and some people simply need and desire more. It's simply like that – reasons off course differ. Some need / want more options to boost the Chi Power because of having severe health issues, long-term disease or because of different other reasons. Examples I can give are professional MMA fighters and other Martial Artists, triathlon runners, CEO's and managers, sales representatives and simply people who are under huge amount of physical and mental stress – they need and ask for more. Because you may be one of them I have turned the complete Chi Meridian stretching exercise program in to a book named Total Chi Fitness. Again, this program you have to consider ONLY if you feel you 'need more' and you have more time to dedicate. Exercises in Total Chi Fitness are simple and not difficult to learn or perform (like in this book you have explanations, photos and I prepare even Videos) so there is no problem to learn them. However you need bit more time for doing them, that is the fact – more power calls for more efforts = more time. One round of Total CHI Fitness (www.amazon.com/dp/B00BZG7NK8) exercises lasts for about 12-15 minutes.

CONCLUSION

The methods presented in this book (as well as in my other books like above explained Total CHI Fitness, www.amazon.com/dp/B00BZG7NK8) are not products of my creation or speculation. Also, these are not a result of 'experimentation' or anything like that.

Yes, they are presented in a simple way that is really easy to apply. Simple is good – I believe you do have that experience. The potency of these 5-Minute Chi Boost methods has not changed within a few thousand years in any way. In the past, these exercises were given from a master to an advanced disciple. Their originality was very carefully preserved over the centuries.

These methods are therefore not only ancient but more importantly they are free from the modern disease of consumerism. If you give them a chance, they will help you change your life. As much as you use them, they will speak to you more and more.

They will refresh your Chi, give you new energy and power to move fast toward your goals. If you are weak and suffer from a disease, this 5-Minute Chi Boost program will help you become healthy again and keep you from sickness and pain. That is the essence and that is the purpose of this small book, or 'manual' might be more appropriate.

Names and theories are not so important – reality is! I wish you to take on these practices in full and use this manual every day until you learn the process. After a short time, you will only need this manual now and then, as a reminder, which is exactly my intention.

Feel free to contact Sifu William Lee at **sifu.william.lee@gmail.com**

Check out his Amazon profile at www.amazon.com/William-Lee/e/B00DWFOCV8

NEXT STEP

Please, write me an honest review about the book – I truly value your opinion and thoughts and I will incorporate them into my next book, which is already being prepared.

Leave your review of my book on Kindle page at www.amazon.com/dp/B009JFKYGC

THANK YOU!

READ MORE BY SIFU LEE

Total Chi Fitness
Healing Chi Meditation
T.A.E. Total Attack Elimination
Chi Healing Powers Book Set
Total Self Defense Book Set
Happy & Gluten Free

And
5-Minute Stress Management

Or Get the Best Deal on Sifu Lee's Packages

Chi Healing Powers Book Set
Total Self Defense Book Set

Copyright and Disclaimer

The author and publishers of this book do not dispense medical advice nor prescribe to the use of any technique or treatment for health disorders and any sort of medical problems without the advice of a medical professional, either directly or indirectly. It is the intention of this book to only offer information of a general nature. Any specific problems should be referred to your doctor. If you choose to use this information for yourself then the author and publisher assume no responsibility whatsoever.